Table of contents

Introduction to Bland diet

A bland diet can be used alongside lifestyle changes to help address the symptoms of ulcers, heartburn, GERD, nausea, and vomiting. You may also need a bland diet after stomach or intestinal surgery.A bland diet includes low fiber foods that have a soft consistency and are gentle on the digestive system. Bland diets are also known as soft diets, low residue diets, and gastrointestinal soft diets.

A doctor might recommend a bland diet for people experiencing gastrointestinal inflammation from infections, diverticulitis, or the flares of a chronic condition, such as Crohn's disease or ulcerative colitis.

People with other gastrointestinal conditions, including acid reflux and peptic ulcers, may also benefit from a bland diet.

As well as specific food recommendations, people following a bland diet may also have to eat smaller meals more frequently, eat more slowly, and avoid lying down soon after eating.

In this book, learn about the food options for people following a bland diet, how it works, and recent research into the topic.

Self-care

A bland diet includes foods that are soft, not very spicy, and low in fiber. If you are on a bland diet, you should not eat spicy, fried, or raw foods. You should not drink alcohol or drinks with caffeine in them.

Your health care provider will tell you when you can start eating other foods again. It is still important to eat healthy foods when you add foods back in. Your provider can refer you to a dietitian or nutritionist to help you plan a healthy diet.

Foods you can eat

Foods you can eat on a bland diet include:

• Milk and other dairy products, low-fat or fat-free only

• Cooked, canned, or frozen vegetables

• Potatoes

• Canned fruit as well as apple sauce, bananas, and melons

• Fruit juices and vegetable juices (some people, such as those with GERD, may want to avoid citrus and tomato)

• Breads, crackers, and pasta made with refined white flour

• Refined, hot cereals, such as Cream of Wheat (farina cereal)

• Lean, tender meats, such as poultry, whitefish, and shellfish that are steamed, baked, or grilled with no added fat

• Creamy peanut butter

• Pudding and custard

• Graham crackers and vanilla wafers

• Popsicles and gelatin

• Eggs

• Tofu

• Soup, especially broth

• Weak tea

Foods to Avoid

Some foods you may want to avoid when you are on a bland diet are:

• Fatty dairy foods, such as whipped cream or high-fat ice cream

• Strong cheeses, such as bleu or Roquefort cheese

• Raw vegetables and salads

• Vegetables that make you gassy, such as broccoli, cabbage, cauliflower, cucumber, green peppers, and corn

• Dried fruits

• Whole-grain or bran cereals

• Whole-grain breads, crackers, or pasta

• Pickles, sauerkraut, and other fermented foods

• Spices and strong seasonings, such as hot pepper and garlic

• Foods with a lot of sugar in them

• Seeds and nuts

• Highly seasoned, cured or smoked meats and fish

• Tough, fibrous meats

• Fried foods

• Alcoholic beverages and drinks with caffeine in them

You should also avoid medicine that contains aspirin or ibuprofen (Advil, Motrin).

Other Diet Tips

When you are on a bland diet:

• Eat small meals and eat more often during the day.

• Chew your food slowly and chew it well.

• Stop smoking cigarettes, if you smoke.

• DO NOT eat within 2 hours of your bedtime.

• DO NOT eat foods that are on the "foods to avoid" list, especially if you do not feel well after eating them.

• Drink fluids slowly.

What can I eat?

Everyone's needs are different, so you may want to discuss your dietary choices with your doctor or a dietitian. They can provide additional input based on your specific diagnosis and lifestyle.

Unless you have a preexisting food allergy or intolerance, commonly recommended foods on the bland diet include:

Low-fat dairy

Low-fat or fat-free milk, yogurt, and mildly flavored cheeses, such as cottage cheese, are all good options. Be careful, though. Lactose intolerance and milk protein intolerance are common reasons for GI discomfort in some people. And many experts recommend eliminating dairy to help treat peptic ulcers.

Certain vegetables

Vegetables you should eat include:

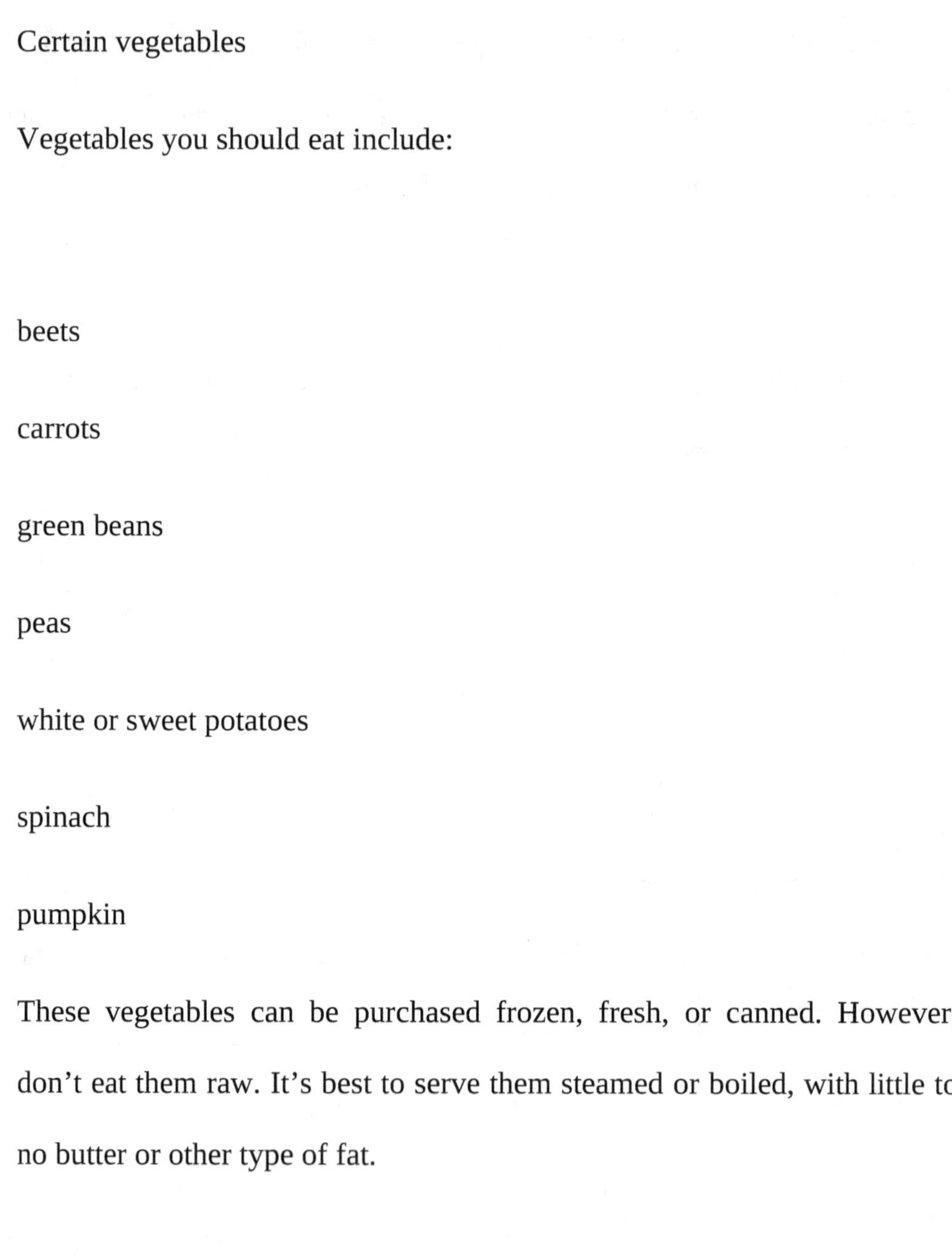

beets

carrots

green beans

peas

white or sweet potatoes

spinach

pumpkin

These vegetables can be purchased frozen, fresh, or canned. However, don't eat them raw. It's best to serve them steamed or boiled, with little to no butter or other type of fat.

Some people can tolerate lettuce and other salad greens in moderation. It's best to exclude vegetables that cause gas, such as those from the cruciferous family. These include broccoli, kale and Brussels sprouts, among others.

Low-fiber fruits

Cooked or canned fruits that aren't fibrous or seeded are generally approved for a bland diet. These include bananas and melon. Avocados may also be tolerated well, even though they're higher in fiber.

Processed grains

White bread products, seedless rye, and refined wheat products may be good choices. However, some people have worsened digestive symptoms when they eat gluten-containing grains.

If you do not have an intolerance to gluten, then you can also enjoy:

plain soda crackers

soft white pasta

cooked cereals, such as cream of wheat, processed oatmeal (not steel-cut or high-fiber), and farina

cold cereals that are low in sugar

Poultry, eggs, and fish

Lean protein sources are safe to eat as long as they're prepared with mild seasonings and little to no fat. These include:

skinless chicken

fish, such as salmon and trout

shellfish, such as shrimp, lobster, and crab

eggs

silken tofu

Other food items

Cream-based soups or clear broths are excellent choices, provided their ingredients are on the list of foods you can eat.

Chamomile tea, with or without honey, can be a soothing drink choice.

Dessert foods, such as vanilla pudding, marshmallows, and plain cookies should only be eaten sparingly because added sugar can worsen symptoms.

Creamy peanut butter, jelly, and jam without seeds are all good options for spreading on bread.

Many seasonings may be irritating to the stomach, but you can experiment with basil, parsley, salt, and other mild flavorings to determine which ones you can tolerate.

High-fat dairy foods and strongly-flavored cheeses should be avoided. These include:

whole milk

whipped cream

ice cream

Monterey Jack cheese

bleu cheese

Roquefort cheese

Also, dairy triggers symptoms in some people, so avoid dairy altogether if this is you.

Certain vegetables

Some vegetables are notorious for producing gas. These include:

cruciferous types, such as Brussels sprouts, broccoli, and cauliflower

onion

garlic

peppers

cabbage

Tomatoes and tomato products are highly acidic and should be avoided.

Seeded and acidic fruit

In general, if fruit has skin or tiny seeds, it has too much fiber for a bland diet. Also, the acidity of some of the fruits may trigger heartburn in some people.

Fruits to avoid include:

all berries

grapes

prunes

oranges

lemons

limes

grapefruits

Most dried fruits and fruit juices should be eliminated, as well.

Whole grains

High-fiber, whole grain foods should be avoided if you are following a

low-fiber or low-residue diet, which is sometimes recommended as part of

a bland diet. Also, gluten may be a trigger for some people, so avoiding all

forms of wheat, rye, and barley may be beneficial.

Avoid these:

sprouted wheat bread

grain breads

whole wheat pasta

any product with added fiber, such as cereal

Fatty meats, poultry, beans, and fish

Lentils and dried or canned beans of all types can generate gas. Beef,

chicken with the skin on, and fried fish may also irritate your gut.

Avoid eating fatty, greasy, or fried protein sources of any kind, as well as processed deli meats. You should also avoid prepared foods, such as beef or chicken tacos, chili, or meat sauce.

Other food items

All types of alcoholic drinks can be irritating to the stomach. So can caffeinated beverages, such as coffee, tea, and soda.

Many dressings and sauces, such as mustard, ketchup, salad dressing, and horseradish, are best left on the shelf.

The following may also make your symptoms worse:

fatty desserts, such as cheesecake and dark chocolate

olives

popcorn

granola

nuts

Bland Diet Recipes

A bland diet — foods that are soft, not spicy, and low in fat and fiber —

can help with nausea, vomiting, diarrhea, and gas after stomach or intestinal surgery. Avoiding gas-producing foods such as cruciferous vegetables is also recommended.

Once you've prepped the vegetables, this White Winter Minestrone Soup goes fast yet tastes as though it has been cooked for hours. It tastes even better the next day. I tend to like my...

Ingredients

3 tablespoons olive oil

1 clove garlic, chopped

1 medium onion, chopped

3 carrots, cut into a large, ½ inch dice

1 stick celery, cut into ½ inch slices (optional)

½ teaspoon dried sage

1 sprig thyme or winter savory, chopped

1 bay leaf, broken

⅓ cups hulled pearl barley

½ small head of Savoy cabbage, cored and cubed (about 1 pound)

2 tablespoons flat-leaf parsley, chopped

Parmesan rind, plus more for grating (optional)

6 to 8 cups of stock or water, or to taste

1 (14 ounce) can of water-cooked Cannellini, Borlotti or Great Northern beans, drained and rinsed or 2 cups home-cooked Cranberry, Northern or Cannellini beans in their broth

Salt and pepper, to taste

Directions

Heat the olive oil in a large saucepan or soup pot on medium-high heat. Add garlic. Fry until it turns to a light gold.

Add the onions, carrots, celery, sage, thyme, and bay leaf. Sauté for a minute. Cover and turn the heat to medium-low. Sweat the vegetables for about 10 minutes, until they soften. Stir from time to time. Do not let them stick and burn!

Add the pearl barley and cabbage. Mix well with the other vegetables. Cover again and sweat for another 3-5 minutes or until the cabbage begins to soften. Add the parsley and cook for another minute or so. Add the stock and Parmesan rind and bring the soup to a boil over a high heat. Cover, turn the temperature to low and simmer gently for 25 minutes, or until the barley is nearly cooked.

Add the beans. If home cooked, add their liquid, too. Bring back to a simmer. Cover and cook for another 10 minutes. Discard bay leaf. Dice the Parmesan rind and return it to the pot. Adjust seasoning and grind a little black pepper on top. Serve with freshly grated Parmesan chees.

Clock Icon for Prep Time20 min prep

Person Icon for Serving Size12 servings

Carrot Icon for Number of Ingredients Size10 ingredients

These Pumpkin Scones are the perfect addition to any fall day. With a cup of coffee in the morning or as a sweet afternoon treat, they are sure to impress – even those that...

Ingredients

2 cups all purpose flour

½ cup granulated sugar

2 teaspoons baking powder

¼ teaspoon baking soda

½ teaspoon ground nutmeg

¾ teaspoon ground cinnamon

¼ teaspoon ground clove

¾ cup unsalted butter, chilled and diced

½ cup canned pumpkin puree

¼ cup plus 1 tablespoon buttermilk

Missing an Ingredient?

Visit our ingredient substitution guide.

Nutrition Facts

Calories 217 cals

Fat 12 g

Saturated Fat   7 g

Polyunsaturated Fat   1 g

Monounsaturated Fat 3 g

Carbohydrates   26 g

Sugar 9 g

Fiber 1 g

Protein3 g

Sodium102 mg

Directions

Preheat oven to 400 degrees. Line a baking sheet with parchment paper.

In a large mixing bowl, combine flour, sugar, baking powder, baking soda, nutmeg, cinnamon, and cloves.

Cut butter into dry ingredients. The butter should be the size of peas in the flour mixture, and look like a coarse meal.

Make a well in the center of the flour and butter. Add the pumpkin and buttermilk to the center of the well. With a spatula, fold the wet ingredients into the dry ingredients being careful not to over-mix.

Once dough is formed, pour onto floured service and shape in a rectangle that is about an inch thick. Using a floured knife, cut rectangle into 10-12 triangles and put on a piece of parchment paper. Chill scones for 20 minutes.

Bake scones for 10-12 minutes, or until golden brown

Lemon-Soy Baked Tofu Steaks

20 min prep

8 servings

9 ingredients

This delicious lemon-soy baked tofu recipe uses a Westernized version of a traditional Japanese teriyaki marinade. For really tasty tofu, the best way is to simply bake the tofu covered in marinade instead of marinating it before cooking. It is important to take the time to press the excess water out of the tofu so that it takes up as much of the marinade as possible during cooking, and doesn't dilute the marinade.

Ingredients

2 blocks of firm tofu, sliced into ½-inch thick slices.

Marinade:

⅔ cup soy sauce

2 teaspoon lemon, grated and zested

4 tablespoons lemon juice

2 tablespoons balsamic vinegar

2 teaspoons sugar

4 tablespoons olive oil (See Chef Tips if on a Bland Diet)

2 cloves garlic, crushed and sliced

2 tablespoon chopped fresh herbs, tarragon, rosemary or thyme (Optional)

Nutrition Facts

Calories

199 cals

Fat

14 g

Saturated Fat

2 g

Polyunsaturated Fat

5 g

Monounsaturated Fat

7 g

Carbohydrates

7 g

Sugar

2 g

Fiber

2 g

Protein

15 g

Sodium

1186 mg

*per serving

Directions

Lay the tofu out on a board or tray lined with paper towels or a clean tea towel. Cover with more paper. Lay a wooden cutting board or other weight on top to press out the excess moisture so that the marinade won't be diluted. (I often use wine or water bottles as weights.) This will take about 30 minutes. It's best to do this near the sink. You will be amazed by how much water comes out.

Preheat the oven to 400 degrees.

Put all the ingredients together in a saucepan, except the herbs. Bring to a boil. Take it off the heat immediately and cool. Add the herbs once the marinade is off the heat.

Once the tofu is drained, pat the slices dry. Spoon a little marinade onto a lightly greased baking dish and lay the tofu slices over it, side by side in a single layer. Pour the rest of the marinade over them. Bake uncovered for 25 minutes, turning the slices over about halfway through. The tofu should be brown and almost dry, and any remaining marinade thick and syrupy. Serve immediately!

Honey Sriracha Tofu & Cauliflower

(5 votes, average: 4.40 out of 5)

30 min prep

3 servings

There is a lot of fear of soy products because of their supposed association with breast cancer, but studies show that they have a protective benefit against breast cancer. In fact, in countries like Japan and China, where soy intake is the highest, the incidence of breast cancer is the lowest. Get all the nutritional benefits of whole soy products like tofu in this mouthwatering dish infused with some of the best Asian-inspired flavors.

READ LESS

Print Recipe

Ingredients

14 ounces of firm tofu, drained, patted dry, and chopped into bite-sized pieces

2 tablespoons soy sauce, divided

4 tablespoons sesame oil, divided

1 head of cauliflower, cut into florets

1-2 tablespoons Sriracha (depending on spice-level desired)

1 tablespoon honey

1 clove garlic, diced

1 tablespoon fresh grated ginger

Zest and juice of 1 orange (can also substitute lemon or lime)

2 teaspoons corn starch

2 tablespoons scallions, chopped

1 cup brown rice, prepared

1 tablespoon sesame seeds

Missing an Ingredient?

Visit our ingredient substitution guide.

Nutrition Facts

Calories

702 cals

Fat

34 g

Saturated Fat

5 g

Polyunsaturated Fat

15 g

Monounsaturated Fat

11 g

Carbohydrates

78 g

Sugar

13 g

Fiber

10 g

Protein

31 g

Sodium

663 mg

*per serving

Directions

Pre-heat oven to 400F

Add chopped and drained tofu to a medium bowl and add 1 tablespoon of soy sauce and 2 tablespoons of sesame oil to marinate for 30 minutes.

Once the tofu is marinated, add the cauliflower florets and the remaining 2 tablespoons of sesame oil, mix to combine

On a parchment or foil lined baking sheet, spread the tofu and cauliflower out evenly. Roast in a pre-heated oven for 20 to 30 minutes, until desired crispiness is achieved.

While the tofu and cauliflower roast, make the sauce: add remaining 1 tablespoon of soy sauce, sriracha, honey, garlic, ginger, orange zest, orange juice to a pan or skillet on medium heat. Stir to combine, then whisk in the corn starch to thicken the sauce.

Once the tofu and cauliflower are removed from the oven, add to the sauce. Mix gently to combine. Toss with chopped scallions.

Serve over brown rice. Top with sesame seeds.

Peanut Butter & Banana Smoothie

5 min prep

1 servings

This smoothie is a real treat when you need something satisfying and soothing — plus it's incredibly easy to make. It's also a delicious vehicle for sneaking in some nutrient-rich leafy greens.

Ingredients

½ cup fat-free milk

½ cup plain non-fat Greek yogurt

1 tablespoon peanut butter

2 cups fresh spinach

1 medium banana

Nutrition Facts

Calories

332 cals

Fat

9 g

Saturated Fat

2 g

Polyunsaturated Fat

2 g

Monounsaturated Fat

4 g

Carbohydrates

44 g

Sugar

27 g

Fiber

6 g

Protein

22 g

Sodium

169 mg

Directions

Combine ingredients in a blender and blend until smooth.

Coconut Cardamom Popsicles

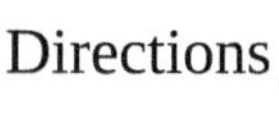 (2 votes, average: 5.00 out of 5)

10 min prep

10 servings

6 ingredients

When the weather warms up or you're in need of a cooling treat while in treatment, you'll want to have these easy-to-make popsicles at the ready. Bananas and coconut offer up a dense source...

READ MORE

Print Recipe

____

Ingredients

1 (14 ounces) can full-fat coconut milk, unsweetened

2 bananas, peeled and frozen

⅓ cup coconut water

¼ cup honey

1 teaspoon ground cardamom

3 tablespoons chia seeds

Missing an Ingredient?

Visit our ingredient substitution guide.

Nutrition Facts

Calories

144 cals

Fat

10 g

Saturated Fat

8 g

Polyunsaturated Fat

1 g

Monounsaturated Fat

1 g

Carbohydrates

15 g

Sugar

10 g

Fiber

2 g

Protein

2 g

Sodium

15 mg

*per serving

Directions

Blend all ingredients in a blender until creamy and smooth.

Pour the blended mixture into popsicle molds and freeze until firm and completely frozen. Enjoy!

Miso Polenta

This creamy polenta manages to still taste utterly delicious and rich without the addition of any dairy. Thanks to umami-rich miso paste and a couple of dried spices we all have in our cupboards, you can transform a simple bowl of food into something spectacular.

Ingredients

4¼ cups water

1 cup polenta

1 tablespoon plus 2 teaspoons miso paste

1/8 teaspoon garlic powder

1/8 teaspoon ground ginger

2 green onions, chopped, to garnish (optional)

Sesame seeds, to garnish (optional)

Directions

In a medium saucepan, bring water to a boil.

Add polenta gradually and whisk until there are no lumps. Lower the heat to low and cook, uncovered, until the mixture thickens, about 20 to 25 minutes. It is important to stir the polenta every five minutes or so to ensure that the bottom of the pan does not burn.

Turn off the heat and add the miso, garlic powder, and ground ginger. Whisk to combine. Serve immediately and garnish with green onions and sesame seeds, if using.

Chicken & Shrimp Jambalaya

Thanks to a couple of minor recipe tweaks and the addition of trusted flavor bombs like Cajun seasoning and hot sauce, this is a healthier twist on a Southern classic that is sure to be your favorite comfort meal.

Ingredients

12 ounces frozen medium shrimp, peeled and deveined

1 teaspoon kosher salt

1 teaspoon of black pepper

2 tablespoons Cajun seasoning, plus

1/2 teaspoon Cajun seasoning, divided

2 tablespoons of extra virgin olive oil

1 medium green bell pepper, diced

1 medium red bell pepper, diced

1 medium yellow onion, diced

2 ribs of celery, diced

4 chicken thighs, boneless and skinless, cubed

1 (14.5 ounces) canned diced tomatoes

2 teaspoons hot sauce

2 teaspoons Worcestershire sauce

1 cup uncooked wild rice

2½ cups chicken stock

2 bay leaves

Directions

Place shrimp in a bowl and season with ¼ teaspoon of salt, ¼ teaspoon of pepper, and ½ teaspoon of Cajun seasoning. Set aside.

In a large pot, warm olive oil on medium heat. Add diced bell peppers, onions, and celery for 10 minutes until onions are translucent. Add remaining salt and pepper and stir to incorporate.

Add the cubed chicken and sauté until chicken browns on all sides, about 8-10 minutes. Add tomatoes, mix, and cook until tomato mixture slightly darkens in color. Add remaining Cajun seasoning, hot sauce, and Worcestershire sauce and stir to combine.

Add wild rice, chicken stock, and bay leaves and simmer for 35-40 minutes, or until rice is tender, but not mushy. Add shrimp and cook until shrimp about 8-10 minutes. Taste and adjust seasonings as needed and serve.

Quinoa & Roast Vegetable Wrap With Spicy Tahini

When getting food on the table feels impossible, you can turn to no-recipe recipes like this one for a filling and nutritious wrap. Feel free to substitute another fiber-rich grain or legume instead of quinoa in this recipe, and get creative and colorful with the kinds of cooked veggies you use — whatever you choose, you'll have a delicious meal ready to eat in no time.

Ingredients

1/4 cup tahini

1/2 cup water, plus more as needed

1/2 lemon, juiced

Salt, to taste

Red pepper flakes, to taste

1 tablespoon chopped fresh parsley

4 whole wheat flour tortillas or other thin flatbread

2 cups quinoa, cooked

3-4 cups cooked vegetable

1 medium avocado, diced

Directions

In a small bowl, whisk together the tahini, water, lemon, salt, red pepper flakes, and parsley. Set aside.

Lay out 4 tortillas or other flatbreads. Add 1/2 cup of quinoa to each wrap, 1 cup of pre-cooked vegetables, and a quarter of an avocado. Drizzle tahini sauce over each wrap.

Enjoy immediately or store in an airtight container in your refrigerator for up to 4 days.

Tahini Shake

This is a naturally sweet and refreshing shake that uses tahini, making it a high-protein treat that's also rich in healthy fats and nut-free. For a dairy-free option, try substituting coconut milk for whole milk.

Ingredients

2 bananas, peeled, sliced, and frozen

1 cup whole milk

¼ tablespoons tahini

4 dates, pitted or 1 tablespoon maple syrup

1½ cups ice

1 teaspoon vanilla extract

1 teaspoon cinnamon (optional)

Directions

Place all ingredients in a blender and blend on high until smooth. Pour into two glasses and garnish with sliced bananas and cinnamon.

Pan-Fried Marinated Tofu

Tofu is a great shapeshifter ingredient and this recipe shows just how versatile it is by pairing it with a Mediterranean flavor profile, perfect for accompanying a bright salad or roast vegetables.

Ingredients

For the marinade

3 tablespoons olive oil

2/3 cup chopped fresh cilantro

1/4 cup chopped fresh mint

1/2 cup lemon juice

6 garlic cloves, minced

1 teaspoon ground cumin

1/2 teaspoon smoked paprika

1/4 teaspoon cayenne (optional)

2 teaspoons agave syrup

1 (1-pound) block extra-firm tofu, cut into 1/2" slices

1 tablespoon olive oil

Cilantro and mint, chopped for garnish

Directions

Add all marinade ingredients and sliced tofu to a resealable plastic bag. Marinate tofu for at least 20 minutes or overnight.

Preheat 1 tablespoon of olive oil in a large saucepan over medium-high heat. When oil starts to ripple, add tofu to pan, being careful not to overcrowd the pan, which can steam instead of fry the tofu. If tofu doesn't sizzle immediately when adding to the pan, remove it and wait another minute.

Cook tofu on both sides until golden, about four minutes on each side. Right before removing tofu from pan, pour in extra marinade from the bag and cook down until it's slightly thickened. Transfer cooked tofu to a plate with sauce and garnished with more fresh herbs. Serve immediately with a crisp salad, roasted vegetables, and/or brown rice.

Spring Watercress Soup

Spring Watercress Soup is easy to make, delicious to eat either hot or chilled, and it's a soup that, once tasted, you will make again and again. It is made with two super greens, watercress and arugula, and you get a protein assist from frozen peas, a pantry staple we all love. The resulting soup has a color that is out of this world, a texture of light cream, and a peppery taste that is mellowed by the sweetness of Vidalia onion and peas. As the ingredients are few, it's a good idea to use a good quality chicken broth or light vegetable broth if you are vegetarian or vegan. Either way, it is a keeper.

Ingredients

1 bunch watercress, well washed

1 tablespoon olive oil

1 small Vidalia onion, in a fine dice

4 cups chicken stock

1 cup frozen peas (see Chef Tips)

4 cups baby arugula

Sea salt to taste

1 tablespoon snipped chives (optional)

2 tablespoons 2% plain Greek yogurt divided (optional)

Whole wheat croutons (optional)

Directions

Take the watercress and separate the thick, tough stems from the leaves. Reserve the leaves and finely dice the stems.

Over a medium high flame, heat the oil in a five quart Dutch oven or other heavy pot. Add the diced watercress stems and the Vidalia onion. Reduce the heat to medium, sprinkle with salt, and sautée until the watercress stems and onion have softened but not taken on any dark color, about five minutes.

Add the stock and bring to a boil over medium-high heat. When the soup boils, reduce heat to medium-low and simmer for 15 minutes.

Add the frozen peas. Cook two minutes or until just soft. Add the reserved watercress leaves and the arugula, stirring until they start to wilt and turn a vivid bright green. Turn off the heat.

Blend the soup with an immersion blender or in batches using a high-speed blender (for safety, fill the vase ½ full each time). Return blended soup to the pan and adjust seasoning as needed. Warm through if serving hot or chill in the refrigerator until cold. Serve with a dollop of yogurt, chopped chives, and croutons, if using.